The Comprehensive Alkaline Cookbook Diet

Delicious Recipes to Supercharge your Energy and Improve your Health

Sam Carter

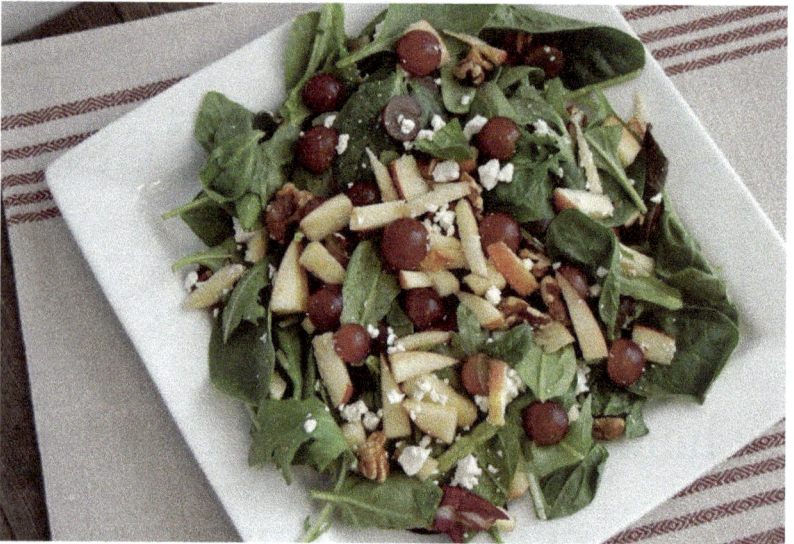

2

contained within this document, including, but not limited to, —
errors, omissions, or inaccuracies.

Table of Contents

Strawberry Coconut Lime Bites

Servings: Makes 6 bites

Total Time: 10 minutes plus 30 minutes chill time

Ingredients

- 6 tablespoons unsweetened, shredded coconut
- 2 teaspoons lime zest
- ⅛ teaspoon Himalayan salt
- ¼ cup coconut butter, melted
- 6 strawberries

Directions

1. On a small plate, combine the shredded coconut, lime zest and salt

2. Take a small spoonful of the coconut butter and press it up against a strawberry. You may need to spread it around the strawberry with your fingers.

3. Roll the strawberry in the coconut lime mixture.

4. Repeat with the remaining strawberries.

5. Set on a large plate and chill in the fridge for at least 30 minutes before serving.

Coconut Chip Bites

Servings: Makes 8 bites

Total Time: 25 minutes

Ingredients

- 1 very ripe banana, mashed

- 2/3 cup unsweetened, shredded coconut

- 1 teaspoon coconut flour

- ¼ teaspoon vanilla extract

- ⅛ teaspoon Himalayan salt

- 1 teaspoon cacao nibs

Directions

1.   Preheat oven to 350°F/175°C. Line a baking tray with parchment paper.

2.   Combine all the ingredients in a large bowl. Mix thoroughly until dough-like texture is created.

3.   Spoon dough into 6 balls on the tray and press down on each ball.

4.   Bake in the oven for 10-15 minutes or until they are lightly browned.

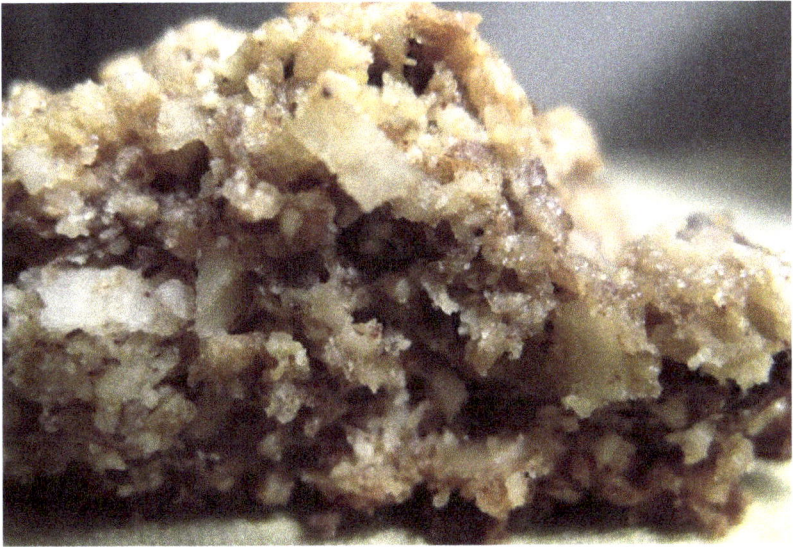

Sweet Potato Orange Cookies

Servings: Makes 12 cookies

Total Time: 35 minutes

Ingredients

- ¾ cup mashed sweet potato

- 1/3 cup quick oats

- 1 tablespoon cashew butter

- 1 egg

- 1 ½ tablespoon honey

- 1 teaspoon orange blossom water

- ¼ teaspoon vanilla

- ¼ teaspoon cinnamon

- ⅛ teaspoon nutmeg

- ¼ teaspoon baking powder

- ¼ teaspoon baking soda

- ⅛ teaspoon Himalayan salt

- 1 teaspoon orange zest

- 1 tablespoon raisins

Directions

1.   Preheat oven to 350°F/175°C. Line a baking tray with parchment paper.

2.   Add all the ingredients, except the raisins to a food processor and blend until combined. Fold in raisins.

3.   Scoop 12 balls of dough onto the baking tray. Flatten with a fork and bake for 20 minutes, flipping once halfway through.

4.   Remove and let cool before serving.

Cashew Coconut Cold Cookies

Servings: Makes 10 cookies

Total Time: 15 minutes plus 30 minutes chill time

Ingredients

- 1/3 cup unsweetened, shredded coconut

- 1/3 cup gluten-free rolled oats

- 1 tablespoon ground flaxseed

- 2 tablespoons cashews, finely ground

- 1/3 cup cashew butter

- 2 tablespoons maple syrup

- 1 teaspoon cacao nibs

- ¼ teaspoon Himalayan salt

Directions

1. In a large bowl, combine all ingredients until a dough forms.

2. Roll 10 pieces of dough into a ball and place on a plate.

3. Chill 30 minutes before serving.

Pumpkin Cups

Servings: 1

Total Time: 5 minutes plus 8 hours chill time

Ingredients

- 1 cup unsweetened almond milk

- 2 tablespoons chia seeds

- ½ teaspoon ground ginger

- ½ teaspoon ground cinnamon

- ¼ teaspoon ground nutmeg

- 1 tablespoon pure maple syrup

- ½ cup pumpkin puree

- ½ teaspoon vanilla extract

- 1 teaspoon flaxseed, ground

- 1 teaspoon unsweetened, shredded coconut

- 1 tablespoon pecans, crushed

Directions

1. Combine all ingredients, except coconut and pecan in a large drinking glass (that has a cover) or a jar. Make sure combined thoroughly.

2. Cover and set in the fridge for at least 8 hours.

3. Garnish with coconut and pecans before serving.

Zippy Ginger Breakfast Bars

Servings: 2 (1 bar each)

Total Time: 10 minutes plus 1 hour chill time

Ingredients

- ¼ cup raw almonds
- ¼ cup raw walnuts
- ½ cup dates, pitted, soaked 10 minutes and then drained
- 1 tablespoon fresh ginger, grated
- ¼ tablespoon cloves
- ¼ teaspoon cardamom
- ¼ teaspoon Himalayan salt

Directions

1. Add all ingredients to a food processor and mix until a sticky dough forms.

2. Shape dough into two equal sized bars and place on a plate in the fridge for at least 1 hour.

Strawberry Toast

Servings: 2

Total Time: 5 minutes

Ingredients

- 2 slices sprouted bread, toasted
- 3 tablespoons almond butter
- 2 tablespoons unsweetened yogurt
- 4 strawberries, hulled and sliced
- ½ teaspoon cinnamon
- 1 tablespoon chia seeds
- 1 tablespoon sunflower seeds

Directions

1. Spread almond butter on each of the slices of toast.

2. Top with yogurt, sliced strawberries, cinnamon, chia seeds and sunflower seeds.

3. Serve immediately.

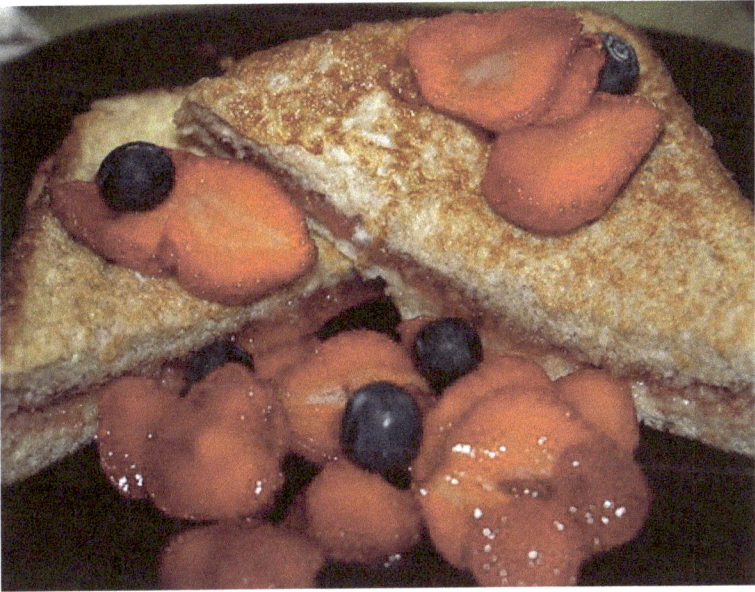

Triple Berry Parfait

Servings: 2

Total Time: 5 minutes

Ingredients

- ½ cup strawberries, hulled, sliced and divided
- ½ cup raspberries, divided
- ½ cup blueberries, divided
- 1 tablespoon chia seeds
- 1 ½ cups unsweetened yogurt
- 2 tablespoons mint, chopped
- 3 tablespoons almonds, slivered

Directions

1. Layer strawberries in the bottom of two tall glasses. Top with half the chia seeds and then a quarter of the yogurt.

2. Top with half raspberries and a half the almonds.

3. Top with half blueberries and half mint.

4. Repeat with remaining glass and ingredients.

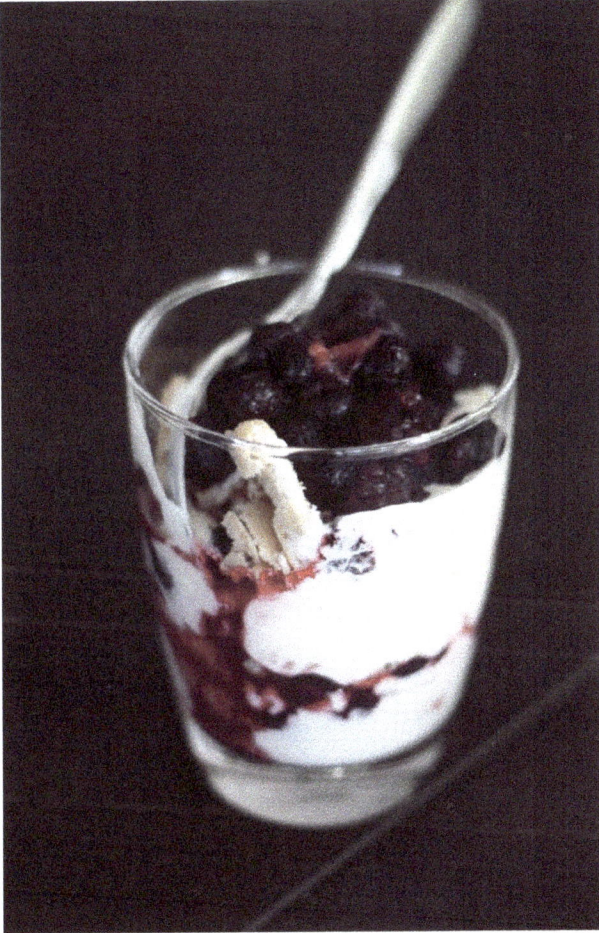

Sweet & Savory Almonds

Servings: 2

Total Time: 30 minutes

Ingredients

- 1 cup raw almonds
- 2 tablespoons raw honey
- 1 tablespoon coconut aminos
- 1 tablespoon tamari
- ½ tablespoon garlic powder
- ½ tablespoon onion powder
- ½ teaspoon celery salt

Directions

1.   Preheat oven to 350°F/180°C. Line baking tray with parchment paper.

2.   Toss all the ingredients in a medium bowl until well coated.

3.   Place almonds on baking tray in an even layer.

4.   Bake in the oven for 25 minutes, stirring every 5 minutes so almonds don't burn.

Plantain Chips

Servings: 2

Total Time: 25 minutes

Ingredients

- 2 large green plantains, sliced
- 1 tablespoon coconut oil
- ½ tablespoon Himalayan salt
- ¼ teaspoon onion powder

Directions

1. Preheat oven to 350°F/180°C. Line baking tray with parchment paper.

2. Toss all the ingredients in a medium-sized bowl until well coated.

3. Add plantain slices to baking tray and bake in the oven for 20 minutes, flipping once after 10 minutes until they are cooked properly to create the "plantain chips."

4. Remove and let cool before serving.

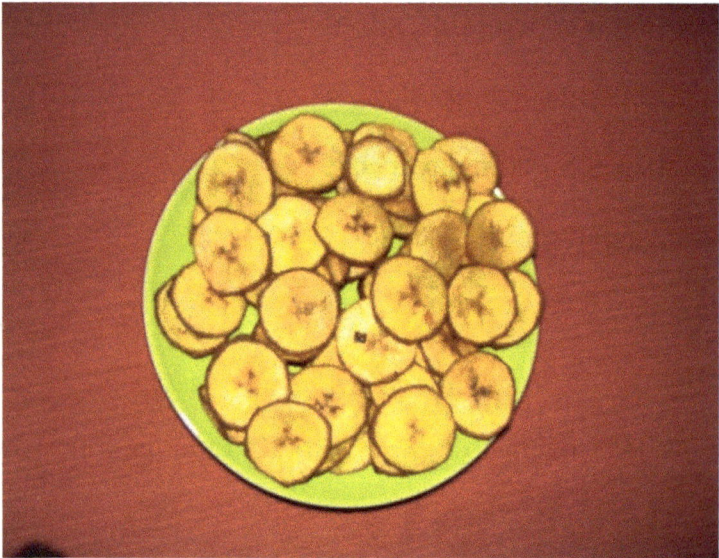

Coconut Figgy Toast

Servings: 2

Total Time: 5 minutes

Ingredients

- 2 sliced sprouted bread, toasted

- 2 tablespoons coconut butter

- 3 fresh figs, sliced

- 1 tablespoon unsweetened, shredded coconut

- 1 teaspoon chia seeds

Directions

1.   Spread coconut butter on top of cooled toast slices. Place figs on top of each slice.

2.   Sprinkle with shredded coconut and chia seeds.

Tamari Pepitas Snack

Servings: 2

Total Time: 25 minutes

Ingredients

- ½ cup pepitas
- 2 tablespoons tamari
- ½ teaspoon coconut aminos
- 1 teaspoon garlic powder
- ½ teaspoon cayenne pepper

Directions

1. Preheat oven to 350°F/180°C. Line baking tray with parchment paper.

2. Toss all the ingredients in a medium-sized bowl until well coated.

3. Add pepitas to baking tray and bake in the oven for 20 minutes, stirring every 5 minutes

4. Remove and let cool before serving. Great to keep in a ziplock bag and snack on throughout the day.

Sweet Roasted Chickpeas

Servings: 2

Total Time: 35 minutes

Ingredients

- 2 cups chickpeas, cooked
- 1 tablespoon coconut oil
- 1 teaspoon cinnamon
- 1 teaspoon nutmeg
- 1 teaspoon coconut sugar

Directions

1. Preheat oven to 400°F/205°C. Toss chickpeas with coconut oil in a small oven proof bowl. Bake in the oven for 30 minutes, mixing frequently.

2. While chickpeas bake, add cinnamon, nutmeg and sugar to a separate medium sized bowl.

3. Remove chickpeas from oven and place immediately in the bowl with the spices. Toss well to coat.

4. Lay on a plate and let cool before serving.

Roasted Broccoli with Tahini Dip

Servings: 2

Total Time: 35 minutes

Ingredients

- 2 cups broccoli, cut into large florets
- 2 tablespoons olive oil
- ½ teaspoon Himalayan salt
- ¼ teaspoon turmeric
- 2 tablespoons tahini
- 1 tablespoon warm water
- ½ tablespoon honey

Directions

1.   Preheat oven to 400°F/205°C. Toss broccoli with oil, salt and turmeric in a small oven proof bowl. Bake in the oven for 30 minutes, turning once.

2.   While broccoli roasts, whisk together the tahini, water, and honey in a small bowl.

3.   Remove broccoli from oven and serve immediately with the tahini dip.

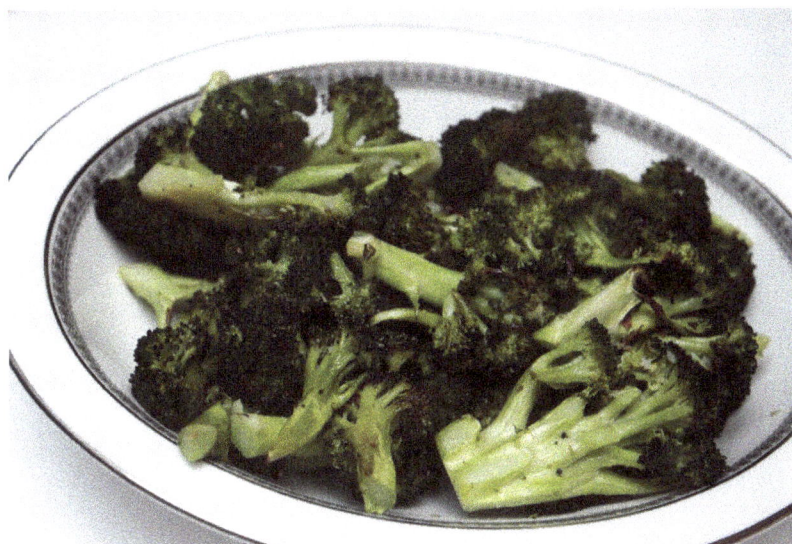

Green Goddess Smoothie

Servings: 1

Total Time: 5 minutes

Ingredients

- 1 avocado
- ½ cucumber
- 1 cup of fresh kale leaves, stems removed
- 1 peeled lime
- ½ cup chopped parsley
- 1 cup water

Directions

1. Place all ingredients into a high speed blender. Pulse a few times to get started then mix on high until smooth.

Spicy & Smooth Green Shake

Servings: 2

Total Time: 5 minutes

Ingredients

- 1 cucumber

- 2 tomatoes

- 1 avocado

- 1 cup spinach leaves

- 1 lime, juiced

- ½ jalapeno, seeded

- ¼ teaspoon red pepper flakes

- ½ cup water

- 1 teaspoon spirulina powder

Directions

1. Combine all ingredients in a blender and combine until smooth. Add more if too thick.

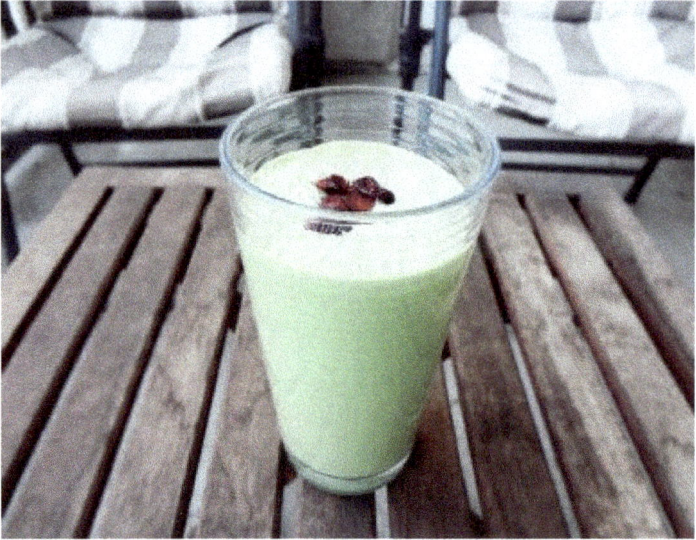

Tropical Smoothie

Servings: 2

Total Time: 5 minutes

Ingredients

- 1 cup pineapple, diced
- 1 cup watermelon, diced
- 2 limes, juiced
- ½ cup cauliflower florets, steamed
- ½ cup cilantro, chopped
- ½ cup coconut water

Directions

1. Place all ingredients in a blender and blend until smooth.

Ginger Blast Smoothie

Servings: 2

Total Time: 5 minutes

Ingredients

- 2 cucumbers, roughly chopped

- 1 lemon, juiced

- 1 lime, juiced

- 2 inch piece of ginger, peeled and sliced

- 2 cups spinach

- 1 apple, cored and roughly chopped

- 1 cup water

- 2 teaspoons chia seeds

Directions

1.   Place all ingredients except the chia seeds in a blender and blend until smooth. Stir in chia seeds and serve.

Spicy Golden Tea

Servings: 2

Total Time: 10 minutes

Ingredients

- 16 ounces water
- 1 inch of fresh turmeric root, peeled and diced small
- 1 inch of fresh ginger root, peeled and diced small
- 2 lemon slices (do not boil, add to tea before serving)
- 2 teaspoons raw honey
- Pinch black pepper

Directions

1.   Place water, turmeric and ginger in a small saucepan and bring to a boil over medium heat.

2.   Reduce heat and let simmer another 5 minutes.

3.   Pour into glasses and add lemon slices, honey and pepper before serving.

Lemon Basil Zinger

Servings: 2

Total Time: 5 minutes

Ingredients

- 2 small lemons, peeled and seeds removed
- 1 ½ tablespoons of coconut oil
- ½ green apple, cored and chopped
- 3 ½ cups water
- ½ teaspoon Himalayan salt
- 1 teaspoon raw honey
- 3 fresh basil leaves
- 4 - 5 ice cubes
- 2 lemon slices

Directions

1.   Place all ingredients in a blender except the lemon slices and blend until fully combined.

2.   Serve with a fresh lemon slice.

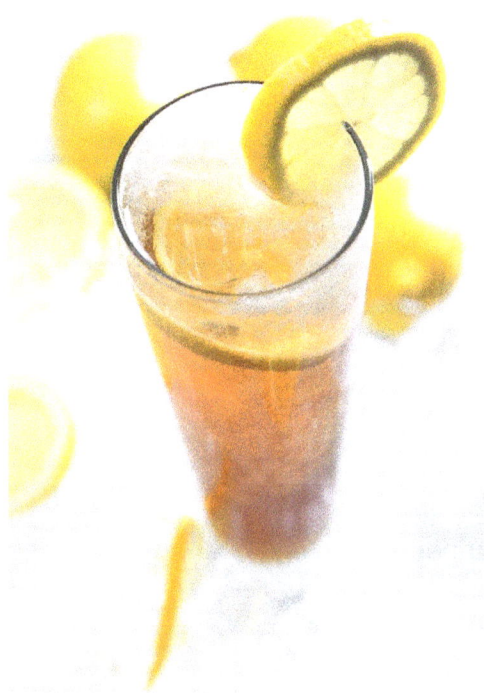

Bloody Mary Shake

Servings: 2

Total Time: 10 minutes

Ingredients

- 1 small cucumber
- 1 celery stalk
- 3 tomatoes
- ½ red bell pepper, seeded and roughly chopped
- 1 garlic clove
- 1 lemon, juiced
- ½ jalapeno, seeded
- ¼ teaspoon pepper
- ½ teaspoon tamari sauce
- ¼ teaspoon cayenne pepper
- 6 - 8 ice cubes
- 4 olives

Directions

1. Place all ingredients in a blender except for the olives and blend until fully combined.

2. Garnish with olives and serve.

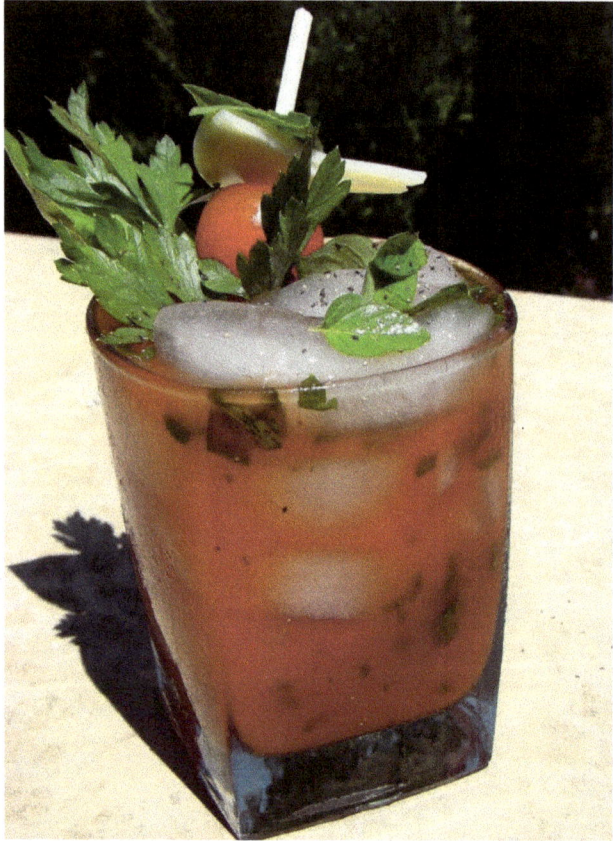

Alkaline Veggie Juice

Servings: 2

Total Time: 5 minutes

Ingredients

- 2 carrots
- 1 cucumber
- ¼ head green cabbage
- 1 cup kale
- ½ lemon
- ½ cup parsley
- 1 inch piece ginger
- 1 inch piece turmeric

Directions

1. Place all ingredients in a juicer and serve immediately.

Fall Lentil Salad

Servings: 2

Total Time: 25 minutes

Ingredients

- 1 small delicata squash, sliced into ½ inch thick slices
- 2 tablespoons olive oil
- 2 teaspoons thyme leaves, chopped
- 1 garlic clove, minced
- 1 tablespoon apple cider vinegar
- 1 tablespoon lemon juice
- ½ tablespoon maple syrup
- ½ teaspoon Himalayan salt
- ½ teaspoon black pepper, crushed
- ½ cup lentils, cooked
- 2 cups spinach, stems removed and thinly sliced
- 2 tablespoons pine nuts, toasted

Directions

1.   Preheat oven to 400°F/205°C. Line a baking tray with parchment paper. In a small bowl, combine the squash, 1 tablespoon olive oil, thyme and garlic. Move the squash to the baking tray and bake in the oven for 20 minutes, flipping once halfway through.

2.   Whisk together the remaining tablespoon olive oil, apple cider vinegar, lemon juice, maple syrup, salt and pepper.

3.   In a large bowl combine the lentils, spinach, baked squash and pine nuts. Drizzle with olive oil mixture, toss to coat and serve immediately.

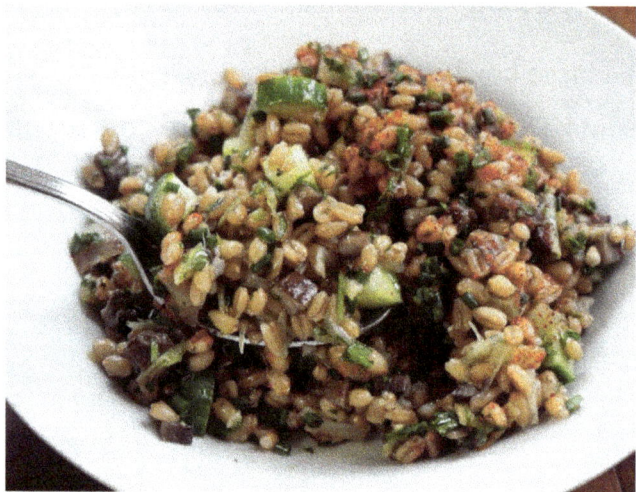

Brown Rice & Sprouts Salad

Servings: 2

Total Time: 5 minutes

Ingredients

- 1 cup brown rice, cooked
- 1 ½ cups of quinoa, cooked
- ½ yellow bell pepper, diced
- 5 cherry tomatoes, halved
- 2 tablespoons cilantro, chopped
- 2 tablespoons parsley, chopped
- 1 cup alfalfa sprouts
- 2 tablespoons almonds, toasted
- 1 tablespoon raisins

Dressing

- 3 tablespoons olive oil
- 1 tablespoon apple cider vinegar
- 1 tablespoon lemon juice
- 1 teaspoon maple syrup
- 1 garlic clove, minced

Directions

1.   In a large serving bowl, place brown rice and top with quinoa, yellow pepper, tomatoes, cilantro, parsley, sprouts, almonds and raisins.

2.   Whisk together Dressing ingredients in a small bowl and pour over the salad.

3.   Toss before serving.

Chopped Beet & Quinoa Salad

Servings: 2

Total Time: 40 minutes

Ingredients

- 2 medium beets, ends cut and halved
- 1 cup quinoa, cooked
- 1 stalk celery, diced small
- ½ head red cabbage, shredded
- 1 garlic clove, minced
- 1 tablespoon apple cider vinegar
- 2 tablespoons olive oil
- ½ teaspoon Himalayan salt
- ¼ teaspoon black pepper, crushed
- ¼ cup fresh mint, chopped
- ¼ cup parsley, chopped

Directions

1. Fill a medium saucepan (fitted with a steamer basket) with water until it reaches halfway. Bring water to a boil over medium

heat and then add beets to the steamer basket. Cover with a lid and reduce heat to low and cook for 30 minutes or until beets are tender.

2.   Remove beet skins by placing in a towel and rubbing off the skins. Chop the cooked beets into a small dice.

3.   In a large bowl, combine quinoa, beets, celery, cabbage, garlic, vinegar, olive oil, salt, pepper, mint and parsley. Combine well and serve immediately.

Sweet Quinoa Salad

Servings: 2

Total Time: 5 minutes

Ingredients

- 3 cups spinach, chopped

- 1 cup quinoa, cooked

- 1 shallot, thinly sliced

- 2 apples, diced

- 2 tablespoons raisins

- 2 tablespoons walnuts, toasted and crushed

- 1 handful sprouts

- 2 tablespoons avocado oil

- ½ lemon, juiced

- ½ teaspoon Himalayan salt

- ⅛ teaspoon cinnamon

- ¼ teaspoon black pepper, ground

Directions

1.   Combine spinach, quinoa, shallot, apples, raisins, walnuts and sprouts in a large bowl.

2.   Drizzle with avocado oil and pour in lemon juice. Add salt, cinnamon and black pepper.

3.   Toss well to combine and serve immediately.

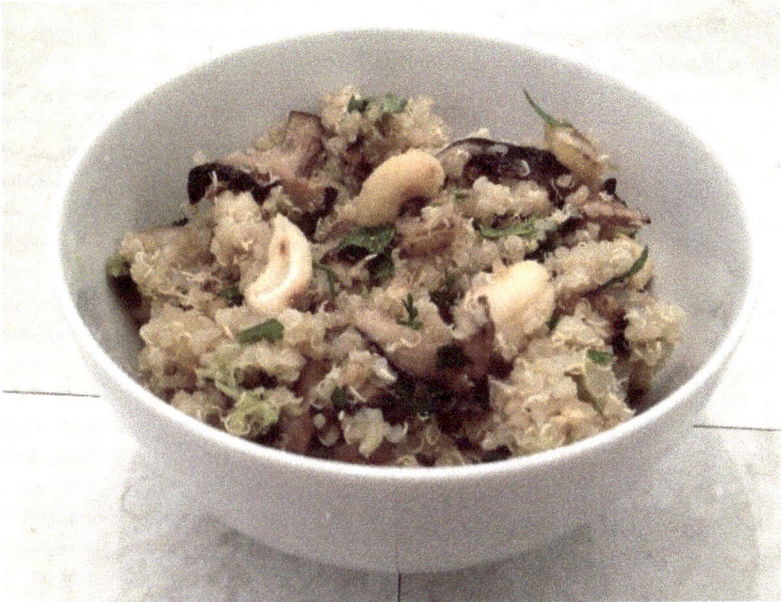

Warm Spinach Salad

Servings: 2

Total Time: 15 minutes

Ingredients

- 1 tablespoon coconut oil

- ½ cup red onion, sliced thinly

- 1 garlic clove, minced

- 5 cherry tomatoes, halved

- 6 cups baby spinach

- ½ teaspoon grated lemon peel

- ½ teaspoon Himalayan salt

- ½ teaspoon black pepper

- ¼ teaspoon cinnamon

- 1 cup brown rice, cooked

- 1 tablespoon pine nuts, toasted

Directions

1.   In a medium skillet over medium heat, melt coconut oil and add onion. Cook 5 minutes and then add the garlic, cooking for an additional 1 minute.

2.   Add in tomatoes and spinach. Season with lemon peel, salt, pepper and cinnamon. Cook for 5 minutes or until spinach is wilted.

3.   Place brown rice in a bowl and top with the spinach and tomato mixture.

4.   Garnish with pine nuts and serve.

Veggie Ramen

Servings: 1

Total Time: 15 minutes

Ingredients

- 1 tablespoon of miso paste
- 1 inch ginger piece, minced
- 1 tablespoon tamari
- ½ lime, juiced
- ½ bell pepper, thinly sliced
- ¼ head of broccoli, cut into small florets
- 1 carrot, spiralized into noodles
- 4 mushrooms, stems removed and sliced
- ½ cup spinach
- ½ zucchini, spiralized
- 3 cups boiling water
- 1 tablespoon cilantro

Directions

1.   In a large bowl that has a lid, add the miso, ginger, tamari, lime juice, bell pepper, broccoli, carrot, mushrooms, spinach and zucchini.

2.   Pour boiling water into the pot, stir well a few times and then place the lid on top.

3.   Let sit 5 minutes and then garnish with cilantro and serve.

Spicy Ginger Salad

Servings: 2

Total Time: 10 minutes

Ingredients

- 3 cups kale
- 1 cup tomatoes, finely diced
- 1 tablespoon parsley, finely chopped
- 1 tablespoon raw sesame seeds
- 1 tablespoon raw pumpkin seeds
- 1 tablespoon almonds
- 1 garlic clove, minced
- ¼ teaspoon lemon zest
- ¼ teaspoon ginger, grated
- ⅛ teaspoon red chili flakes

Dressing

- 3 tablespoons olive oil
- 1 tablespoon lemon juice
- 1 tablespoon apple cider vinegar

- ¼ teaspoon fresh ginger juice

- ½ teaspoon Himalayan salt

- ¼ teaspoon cayenne pepper

- ¼ teaspoon black pepper, crushed

Directions

1.   Make the Dressing by combining the Dressing ingredients in a small bowl until well combined.

2.   In a large bowl, combine the kale, tomatoes, parsley, sesame seeds, pumpkin seeds, almonds, garlic, lemon zest, ginger and chili flakes.

3.   Pour Dressing over the kale and tomato mixture. Let rest 5 minutes before serving.

Curry Squash Soup

Servings: 2

Total Time: 25 minutes

Ingredients

- 1 tablespoon olive oil

- 1 shallot, sliced

- 1 yellow squash, diced

- ½ cup broccoli, cut into florets

- 1 teaspoon ginger, grated

- ½ teaspoon Himalayan salt

- ½ teaspoon black pepper, crushed

- ½ teaspoon cumin

- ½ teaspoon coriander

- ½ teaspoon cardamom

- ½ teaspoon turmeric

- ¼ teaspoon cinnamon

- 1 ½ cups vegetable broth

- ½ cup water

- 1 lemon, juiced

- 1 tablespoon cilantro, chopped

- 1 teaspoon pepitas, toasted

Directions

1.　　Heat oil in a medium-sized pot over medium heat. Add shallot, squash, broccoli, ginger, salt, pepper, cumin, coriander, cardamom, turmeric and cinnamon.

2.　　Sauté 10 minutes until vegetables are softened and then add the broth, water and lemon juice. Let come to a low boil and then reduce heat to low and simmer 10 minutes.

3.　　Let cool 5 minutes and then transfer to a food processor or blender and blend until smooth.

4.　　Top with cilantro and pepitas to serve.

Sweet Potato Nacho Boat

Servings: 2

Total Time: 35 minutes

Ingredients

- 2 sweet potatoes
- ½ tablespoon balsamic vinegar
- ½ teaspoon coconut aminos
- ½ tablespoon apple cider vinegar
- ½ teaspoon cayenne pepper
- ¾ cup tempeh, diced
- 1 cup spinach
- 4 black olives, sliced
- 1 tomato, diced
- 1 shallot, diced
- ½ avocado, diced

Cheese Sauce

- ¼ head of cauliflower, steamed
- ½ cup nutritional yeast
- ½ cup vegetable broth

- 1 garlic clove, minced

- ¼ teaspoon cayenne pepper

- 1 tablespoon white miso

- 1 tablespoon lemon juice

- 1 teaspoon tahini

- ½ teaspoon chili powder

Directions

1. Preheat oven to 400°F/205°C. Line a baking tray with parchment paper. Pierce sweet potatoes with a fork a few times and place on tray. Bake in the oven for 30 minutes.

2. Prepare Cheese Sauce by placing Cheese Sauce ingredients in a food processor or blender and mixing until smooth. Set aside.

3. In a small skillet over medium heat, add balsamic vinegar, coconut aminos, apple cider vinegar and cayenne. Let heat for 3 minutes and then add tempeh, tossing to coat. Cook 5 minutes until tempeh is warm and sauce is slightly reduced.

4. Cut open each sweet potato and add spinach, tempeh, olives, tomato, shallot and avocado. Drizzle cheese sauce on top and serve immediately.

Brussel Sprouts Bowl

Servings: 2

Total Time: 35 minutes

Ingredients

- 1 bunch brussel sprouts, halved

- 1 small red onion, sliced thinly into half-moon shapes

- 2 tablespoons ghee, melted

- 1 cup brown rice, cooked

- ½ cup walnuts, chopped

- 2 tablespoons raisins

- 2 tablespoons pomegranate seeds

- 1 teaspoon Himalayan salt

- 1 teaspoon black pepper

- 1 tablespoon parsley, chopped

Directions

1.   Preheat oven to 400°F/205°C. On a baking tray, place brussel sprouts and red onion. Drizzle with ghee and roast in the oven for 30 minutes or until brussel sprouts are crispy.

2.   Place brussel sprouts, brown rice, walnuts, raisins and pomegranate seeds in a large bowl. Season with salt and pepper.

3.   Garnish with parsley and serve warm.

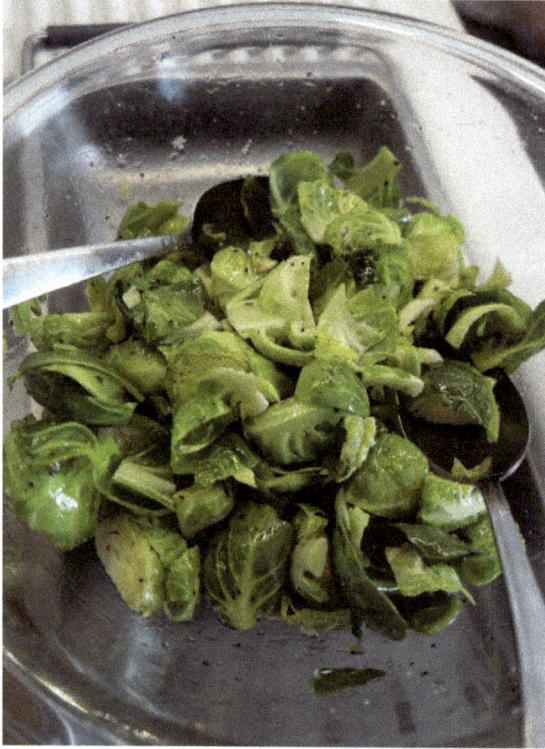

Breakfast Squash Bread

Servings: 2

Total Time: 40 minutes

Ingredients

- 1 cup almond meal
- 1 tablespoon flax meal
- 1/3 cup arrowroot flour
- ½ tablespoon chia seeds
- ½ teaspoon baking soda
- 1 tablespoon dried oregano
- ½ teaspoon Himalayan salt
- 1 egg
- ½ zucchini, finely grated
- ½ yellow squash, finely grated
- 2 tablespoons coconut milk
- 2 tablespoons coconut oil
- ½ teaspoon apple cider vinegar

Directions

1.	Preheat oven to 350°F/180°C. Line a mini loaf tin with parchment paper.

2.	In a medium-sized bowl, combine the almond meal, flax meal, arrowroot, chia seeds, baking soda, oregano and salt.

3.	Beat the egg in a large bowl and add the zucchini, squash, coconut milk, coconut oil and vinegar. Pour the dry ingredients into the large bowl with the wet ingredients and stir until well combined.

4.	Pour mixture into the prepared mini loaf pan and bake in the oven for 20-30 minutes or until lightly golden brown and cooked in the center.

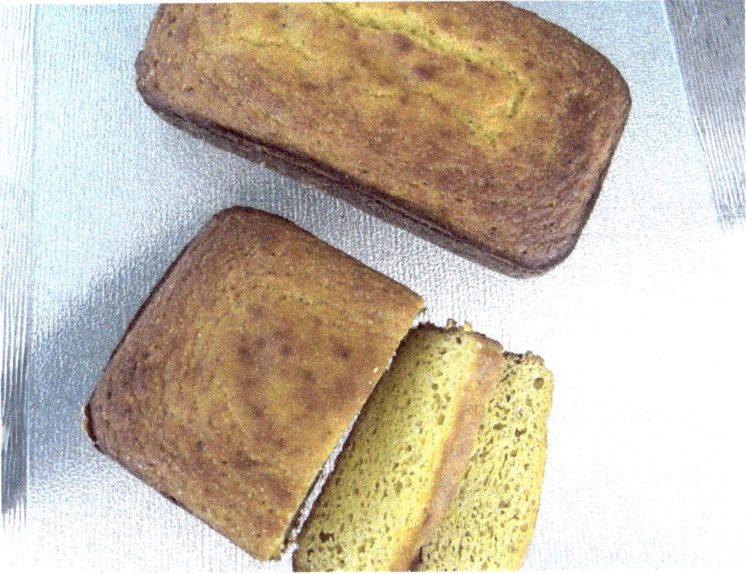

Cherry Almond Bake

Servings: 2

Total Time: 50 minutes plus 30 minutes cooling

Ingredients

- 3 tablespoons unsweetened almond milk

- ¼ cup dates, pitted

- 1/3 cup almond meal

- ¾ teaspoon vanilla extract

- ¼ teaspoon almond extract

- ⅛ teaspoon Himalayan salt

- ¼ cup raw almonds, slivered and divided

- 1 ½ cups fresh cherries, pitted, divided

- 1 cup quinoa, cooked

Directions

1.   Preheat oven to 350°F/180°C and line a small baking dish with parchment paper.

2.   Combine the almond milk, dates, almond meal, vanilla extract, almond extract, salt, half of the almonds and half of the cherries in a food processor or blender.

3.   Add mixture to a large bowl and stir in the quinoa. Pour into prepared baking dish and place remaining cherries and almonds on top.

4.   Bake in the oven for 45 minutes or until lightly browned on top.

5.   Remove from oven and let cool for 30 minutes before cutting into squares and serving.

Salmon & Cabbage Hash

Servings: 2

Total Time: 12 minutes

Ingredients

- 1 tablespoon olive oil

- 1 cup green cabbage, thinly shredded

- 1 cup sweet potato, shredded

- 3 green onions, thinly sliced, divided

- 4 ounces smoked salmon, flaked into bite-size pieces

- ¼ teaspoon black pepper, ground

- 1 tablespoon fresh dill, chopped

Directions

1. In a medium-sized skillet over medium heat, add olive oil, cabbage, sweet potato and half the green onions. Sauté for 8 minutes until cabbage is soft and sweet potato is tender.

2. Add smoked salmon, pepper and dill. Cook 2 minutes.

3. Remove from heat and garnish with remaining green onions before serving.

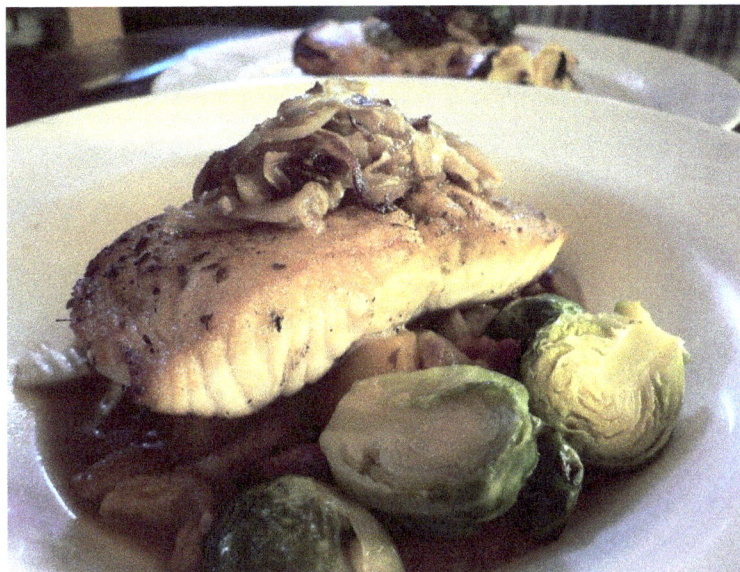

Summer Medley Parfait

Servings: 2

Total Time: 10 minutes

Ingredients

- 1/3 cup raw cashews
- ½ tablespoon raw honey
- ½ teaspoon vanilla extract
- ¼ teaspoon almond extract
- 1 teaspoon lemon juice
- ⅛ teaspoon Himalayan salt
- 1 ½ cups strawberries, hulled, chopped and divided
- ½ tablespoon fresh mint, thinly sliced
- 1 cup honeydew, diced
- 1 teaspoon lemon zest
- 1/3 cup almonds, slivered and toasted

Directions

1.   In a food processor, combine the drained cashews, raw honey, vanilla extract, almond extract, lemon juice and salt. Add

half of the strawberries and pulse until everything is combined thoroughly.

2.   Pour cashew mixture into serving bowls or glasses and top with remaining strawberries, mint, honeydew, lemon zest and almonds.

3.   Serve immediately.

Mexican Breakfast Toast

Servings: 2

Total Time: 5 minutes

Ingredients

- 2 slices sprouted bread, toasted
- 2 tablespoons hummus
- ½ cup spinach, chopped
- ¼ red onion, sliced
- ½ cup sprouts
- 1 avocado, thinly sliced
- ¼ teaspoon Himalayan salt

Spicy Yogurt

- 3 tablespoons unsweetened yogurt
- ½ lime, juiced
- 1 teaspoon cumin
- 1 teaspoon cayenne

Directions

1.   In a small bowl, prepare the Spicy Yogurt by combining all the Spicy Yogurt ingredients and whisking well to combine.

2.   Place toast slices on plates and spread a tablespoon of hummus on each. Place spinach on each slice and then Spicy Yogurt, red onion, sprouts and avocado. Sprinkle each with salt and serve.

Omega- Overnight Oats

Servings: 2

Total Time: 5 minutes

Ingredients

- 1 small ripe banana, mashed

- 1/3 cup rolled oats

- ¾ cup unsweetened almond milk

- ½ teaspoon vanilla extract

- ½ teaspoon cinnamon

- ¼ teaspoon nutmeg

- ⅛ teaspoon Himalayan salt

- 1 tablespoon chia seeds

- 1 tablespoon ground flaxseeds

- 1 teaspoon raw honey

- 1 tablespoon raw almonds, slivered and divided

- ¼ cup blackberries

Directions

1.	Place banana, oats, almond milk, vanilla, cinnamon, nutmeg, salt, chia seeds, flaxseeds, honey and half of the almonds in a medium-sized bowl with a lid or a jar. Stir well to combine and cover.

2.	Leave in the fridge overnight.

3.	When ready to eat, top with remaining almonds and the blackberries.

Broccoli Omelet

Servings: 2

Total Time: 15 minutes

Ingredients

- 12 ounces firm tofu
- 3 tablespoons unsweetened almond milk
- 3 tablespoons nutritional yeast
- 3 tablespoons tapioca starch
- 1 teaspoon Dijon mustard
- ¼ teaspoon turmeric
- ¼ teaspoon black pepper, crushed
- 2 tablespoons green onions

Filling

- 1 cup broccoli, steamed
- 1 shallot, sliced
- 2 tablespoons nutritional yeast

Directions

1.   Combine the tofu, almond milk, nutritional yeast, tapioca, mustard, turmeric and pepper in a food processor or blender until smooth.

2.   Heat a large, nonstick skillet over medium-high heat until very hot. Pour batter into the skillet and let cook for 7 minutes, being careful not to burn.

3.   Place Filling ingredients on one side of the omelet and flip over the other side to cover.

4.   Cook another 3 minutes and then transfer to a plate and garnish with green onions.

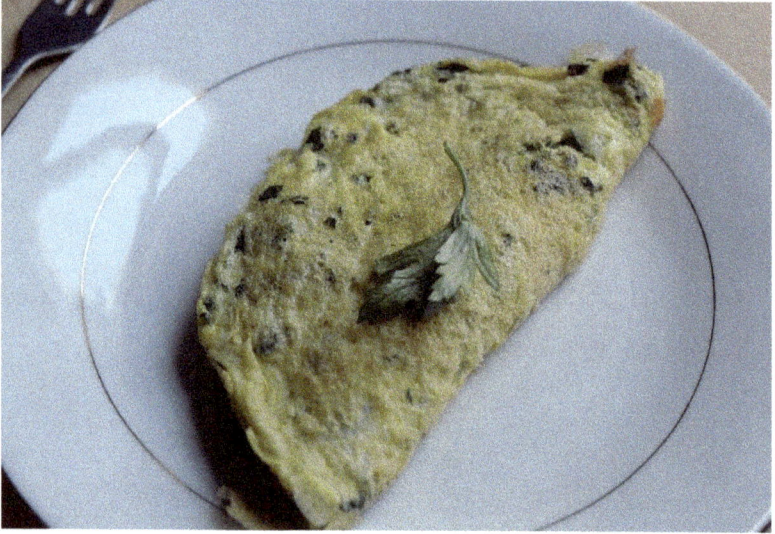

Tofu & Kale Tacos

Servings: 2

Total Time: 12 minutes

Ingredients

- 1 tablespoon coconut oil

- 7 ounces extra-firm tofu, drained

- 2 tablespoons nutritional yeast

- 1 teaspoon onion powder

- ¼ teaspoon turmeric

- 1 tablespoon coconut aminos

- 1 cup kale, thinly sliced

- 5 cherry tomatoes, halved

- 4 corn tortillas, warmed

- 1 tablespoon green onions, sliced

- 1 tablespoon cilantro, chopped

- 1 avocado, sliced

Directions

1. Heat coconut oil in a medium-sized skillet over medium heat. Add tofu, nutritional yeast, onion powder, turmeric and coconut aminos. Cook 5 minutes.

2. Add kale and cherry tomatoes to the skillet and cook another 5 minutes.

3. Remove tofu kale mixture from the stove and divide among the tacos.

4. Top with green onions, cilantro, avocado and serve.

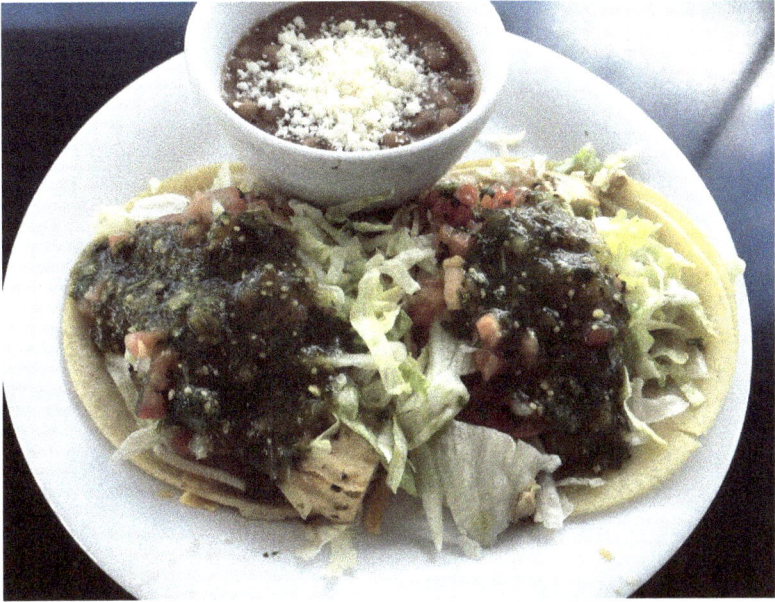

Fruit Porridge

Servings: 2

Total Time: 25 minutes

Ingredients

- ½ cup whole buckwheat
- ½ cup water
- ½ cup unsweetened almond milk
- 1 tablespoon dried apricot, diced
- 2 tablespoons raisins
- 1 cinnamon stick
- ¼ teaspoon nutmeg
- ¼ teaspoon vanilla extract
- 1 teaspoon ground cardamom
- 1 tablespoon pomegranate seeds
- 1 tablespoon walnuts, toasted and crushed

Directions

1.   In a medium saucepan, add buckwheat, water, almond milk, apricot, raisins, cinnamon, nutmeg, vanilla and cardamom.

Bring to a boil and then allow to simmer, stir frequently for 20 minutes or until liquid is absorbed.

2.　　Remove from heat, remove cinnamon stick and garnish with pomegranate seeds and walnuts before serving.

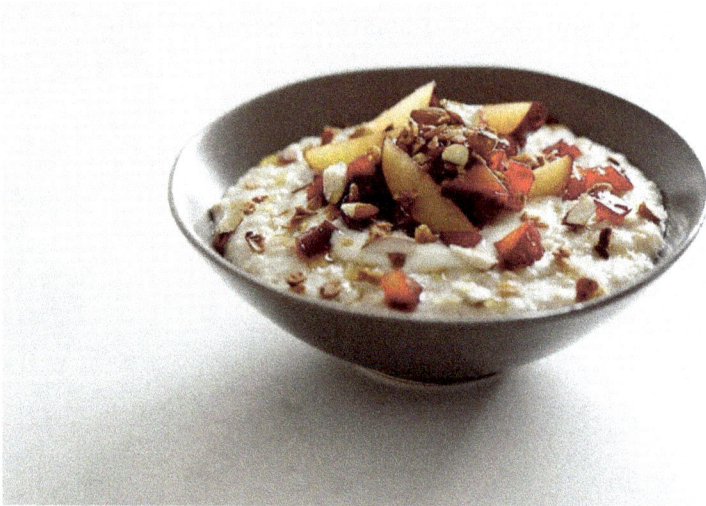

Morning Sweet Bread

Servings: 2

Total Time: 30 minutes

Ingredients

- 1 tablespoon flaxseed, ground
- 3 tablespoons water
- 1 ½ cups almond meal
- 2 tablespoons coconut flour
- 1 teaspoon Himalayan salt
- 2 teaspoon cinnamon
- 1 teaspoon vanilla extract
- 1 teaspoon raw honey
- 1 tablespoon olive oil
- 2 tablespoons raisins
- 1 tablespoon cashew butter, melted
- 1 pear, cored and sliced

Directions

1.   Preheat oven to 350°F/180°C and line bottom of a small glass baking dish with parchment paper.

2.   In a small bowl, mix together the flaxseeds and 3 tablespoons water to from the flaxseeds gel. Set aside and let sit 10 minutes until it forms a gel.

3.   In a large bowl, combine the almond meal, coconut flour, salt, cinnamon, vanilla, honey, flaxseeds gel, olive oil and raisins.

4.   Place dough in the baking dish and press into an even layer. Bake in the oven for 15 minutes.

5.   Remove and let cool. Top with cashew butter and pear slices before serving.

Banana Breakfast Pudding

Servings: 1

Total Time: 5 minutes plus 8 hours chill time

Ingredients

- 1 cup coconut milk
- 1 tablespoon raw honey
- ½ teaspoon vanilla extract
- ¼ teaspoon cinnamon
- ¼ teaspoon nutmeg
- ⅛ teaspoon Himalayan salt
- 2 tablespoons chia seeds
- 1 banana, sliced
- 1 tablespoon walnuts, toasted and crushed
- 1 tablespoon cacao nibs

Directions

1.   In a small bowl or jar with a cover, place coconut milk, honey, vanilla, cinnamon, nutmeg, salt and chia seeds.

2.   Let sit in the fridge, covered, overnight.

3.   In the morning, top with banana, walnuts and cacao nibs before serving.

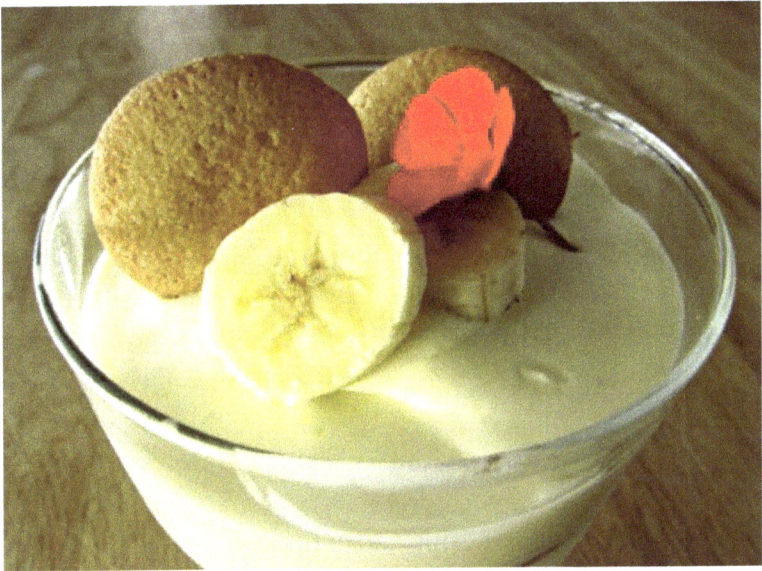

Italian Breakfast Hash

Servings: 2

Total Time: 35 minutes

Ingredients

- 2 sweet potatoes, peeled and cubed into ½ inch pieces
- 2 tablespoons olive oil
- ½ red onion, chopped
- ½ red bell pepper, halved and sliced
- ½ green bell pepper, halved and sliced
- 1 garlic clove, minced
- ½ teaspoon Himalayan salt
- ½ teaspoon black pepper, crushed
- ¼ teaspoon paprika
- 4 fresh sage leaves, thinly sliced
- 1 teaspoon oregano
- ¼ teaspoon red chili flakes
- 1 cup tempeh, crumbled
- 1 tablespoon parsley, chopped

Directions

1.   Place sweet potato cubes in a medium pot over medium-high heat. Bring to a boil and let cook 5 minutes. Potatoes should be tender but not mushy. Drain and set aside.

2.   Heat oil in a large skillet over medium-low heat. Add onion, both bell peppers, garlic and sweet potatoes. Cook 10 minutes, stirring frequently.

3.   Stir in the salt, pepper, paprika, sage, oregano and chili flakes. Cook 2 minutes and then crumble in the tempeh. Cook another 2 minutes and then remove from heat.

4.   Garnish with parsley before serving.

Papaya Breakfast Boat

Servings: 2

Total Time: 5 minutes

Ingredients

- 1 papaya, cut lengthwise in half and seeds removed
- 1 cup unsweetened yogurt
- 1 lime, zested
- 3 tablespoons raw oats
- 1 tablespoon unsweetened shredded coconut
- ½ banana, sliced
- ¼ cup raspberries
- 1 tablespoon walnuts, chopped
- 1 teaspoon chia seeds
- 1 teaspoon raw honey

Directions

1.   Place papaya halves on plates and place yogurt on top of each.

2.   Then top each half with lime zest, oats, coconut, banana, raspberries, walnuts, chia seeds.

3.   Drizzle with honey and serve.

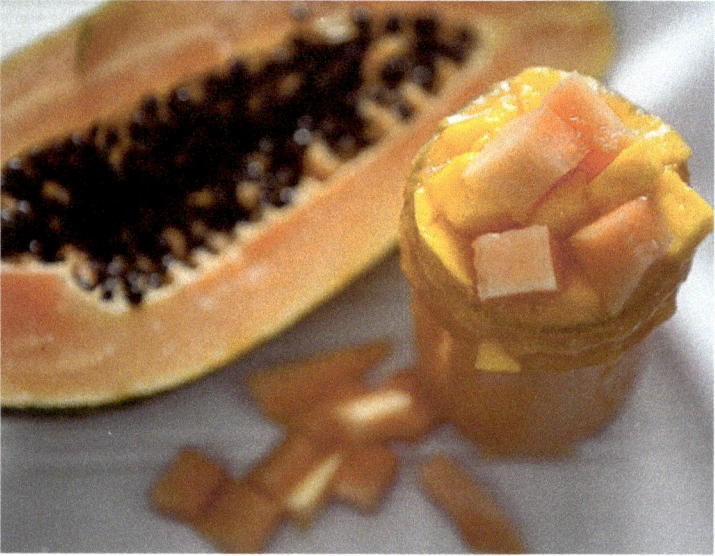

AM Quinoa Cookies

Servings: 2

Total Time: 25 minutes

Ingredients

- ¼ cup almond butter

- 1 tablespoon honey

- ½ medium ripe banana, mashed

- 1 egg, beaten

- ½ teaspoon vanilla

- ¼ teaspoon almond extract

- ¼ cup gluten-free oats

- ¼ cup quinoa flakes

- ½ teaspoon baking powder

- ¼ teaspoon Himalayan salt

- ¼ cup unsweetened, shredded coconut flakes, toasted

- 1 tablespoon chia seeds

- 1 teaspoon flaxseed, ground

Directions

1.   Preheat oven to 350°F/180°C and line a baking tray with parchment paper.

2.   In a large bowl, combine the almond butter, honey, banana, egg, vanilla and almond extract.

3.   In a medium-sized bowl, combine the oats, quinoa flakes, baking powder, salt, coconut flakes, chia seeds and flaxseed.

4.   Add the oat mixture to the almond butter mixture and stir well to combine.

5.   Using 2 tablespoons as a guide, form small balls and place dough onto the baking tray until all dough is used.

6.   Bake in the oven for 15 minutes.

7.   Remove and let cool before serving.

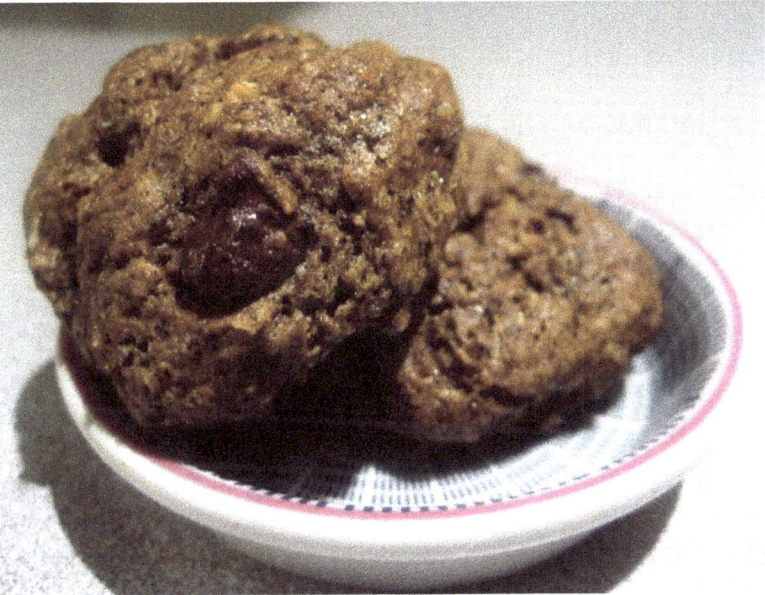

Savory Breakfast Bowl

Servings: 1

Total Time: 20 minutes

Ingredients

- ½ cup rolled oats

- ½ cup unsweetened almond milk

- ½ cup water

- ¼ teaspoon Himalayan salt

- ¼ teaspoon black pepper, crushed

- 1 cup spinach

- 1 tablespoon nutritional yeast

- 1 teaspoon lemon zest

- ½ teaspoon turmeric

- ¼ teaspoon red chili flakes

- 1/3 cup lentils, cooked

- 1 tablespoon green onions, sliced

Directions

1.	In a medium saucepan over medium heat, add oats, almond milk, water, salt and pepper. Bring to a boil and then reduce heat to low and simmer 5-10 minutes or until liquid is absorbed.

2.	Stir in the spinach, nutritional yeast, lemon zest, turmeric, chili flakes and lentils.

3.	Remove from heat and garnish with green onions before serving.

Almond Butter & Jelly Overnight Oats

Servings: 1

Total Time: 10 minutes plus 8 hours chill time

Ingredients

- ½ cup rolled oats
- ¾ cup unsweetened almond milk
- ½ teaspoon vanilla extract
- 1 teaspoon chia seeds
- 1 tablespoon almond butter
- 1 tablespoon sliced almonds
- 4 raspberries, sliced

Raspberry Jam

- ¼ cup raspberries, mashed
- 1 teaspoon honey
- 1 tablespoon chia seeds

Directions

1.   In a small bowl, place the ¼ cup mashed raspberries, honey and 1 tablespoon chia seeds. Combine well and set aside in the fridge for 10 minutes.

2.   Place oats, almond milk, vanilla, chia seeds and 1 tablespoon of raspberry mixture in a small jar and mix well. Cover and let sit in the fridge overnight.

3.   In the morning, add almond butter, sliced almonds and remaining raspberries before serving.

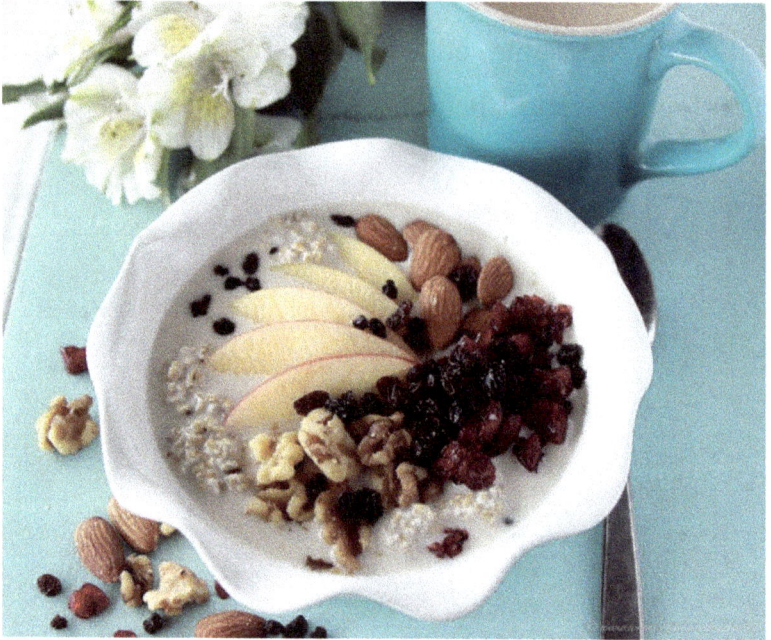

Fruit Skewers

Servings: Makes 4 skewers

Total Time: 10 minutes plus 30 minutes chill time

Ingredients

- 8 raspberries

- 8 pineapple cubes (about ½ inch)

- 8 blueberries

- 8 mango cubes (about ½ inch)

- 8 small mint leaves

- 8 bamboo skewers

Chocolate Sauce

- 2 tablespoons coconut oil, melted

- 1 tablespoon maple syrup

- 2 teaspoons raw cacao powder

Directions

1. Place fruit and mint on the skewers in the desired pattern.

2. Make chocolate sauce by whisking together the coconut oil, maple syrup and cacao powder until smooth.

3.   On a baking tray lined with parchment paper, place fruit skewers.

4.   Drizzle with chocolate sauce and chill 30 minutes in the fridge.

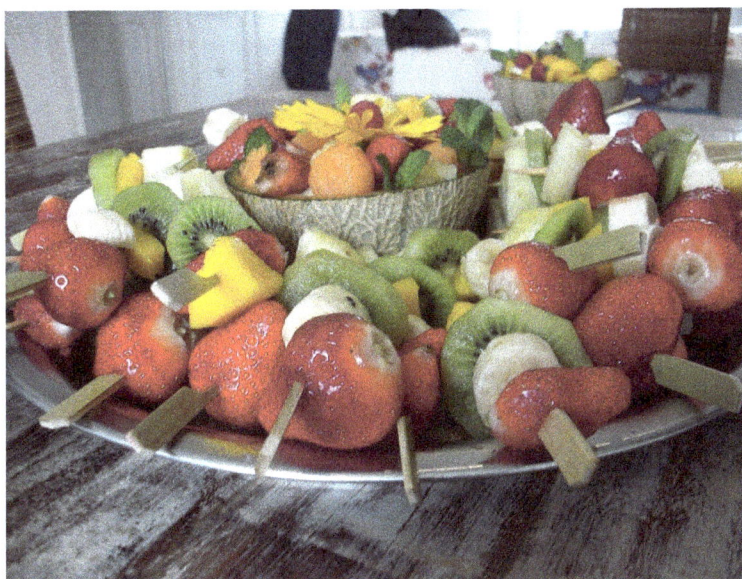

Mint Chocolate Mousse

Servings: 2

Total Time: 5 minutes plus 2 hours chilling

Ingredients

- 1 10 ounce package silken tofu
- 2 teaspoons raw cacao powder
- ½ teaspoon vanilla extract
- ½ teaspoon peppermint extract
- ¼ teaspoon Himalayan salt
- 1 teaspoon raw honey
- 1 tablespoon cacao nibs
- 4 small mint leaves

Directions

1. In a food processor, blend together all ingredients except the cacao nibs and mint leaves until smooth.

2. Pour into two cups and chill in the fridge for 2 hours or until ready to serve. Garnish with cacao nibs and mint leaves before serving.

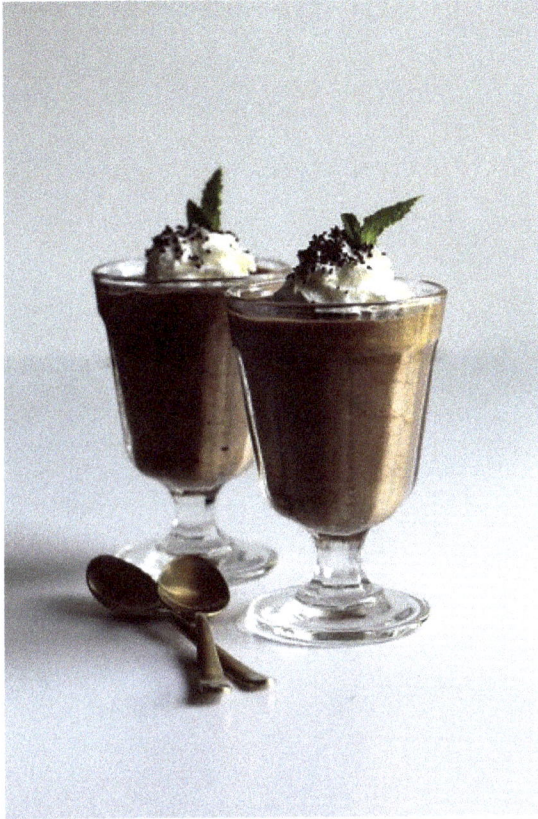

www.ingramcontent.com/pod-product-compliance
Lightning Source LLC
Chambersburg PA
CBHW050754030426
42336CB00012B/1812